Julio Antonio Trillo Granados
Daniel Díaz Plascencia
José Luis Guevara Valdez

Estimation of age in equines by their dentition

Julio Antonio Trillo Granados
Daniel Díaz Plascencia
José Luis Guevara Valdez

Estimation of age in equines by their dentition

Equine dentistry

ScienciaScripts

AGE ESTIMATION IN EQUINES BY DENTITION

POR:

I.Z.P.S. JULIO ANTONIO TRILLO GRANADOS

D. PH. DANIEL DÍAZ PLASCENCIA

D. PH. JOSÉ LUIS GUEVARA VALDEZ

CONTENTS

INTRODUCTION

The horse in the Americas has been of great importance throughout human history. In the mid-16th century, during the time when Hernán Cortés conquered Mexico, the Aztec Indians saw the horse for the first time and were impressed by the imposing, tall animal. When they saw the man on the horse, they thought that the rider and horse were one animal, just like the myth of the centaurs, half man and half horse. The Aztecs' great fear of horses made the conquest of Mexico quick and easy for the Spaniards; this assumes that the horse did not exist in all of America, so we can rule out that the North American Indians were the first tamers of wild horses. However, thousands of centuries earlier there were large herds of horses quite different from today's horses throughout the Americas, but they became extinct and only the fossilised remains were left as evidence.These ancestors of the horses moved towards the south of America, crossing the Panama Canal, populating the entire American continent. It is important to point out that this equine, judging by its fossils, was not similar to today's horse, but resembled donkeys or zebras. Although today's horse has been domesticated in America for many centuries, it is important to emphasise that its ancestors descended from America, as these ancestors crossed the Bering Strait to the north of Asia and from there they spread and populated the whole of Europe, where they evolved into today's horse, which centuries later returned to the American continent with the conquest of Hernán Cortés. As time went by, the natives of North America lost their fear of the horse, domesticating it and using it, as the Spaniards did, for the fight they had with the white man. In these battles they escaped several horses, which were left in complete freedom to later form the great herds of wild horses, the so-called "mustangs". The horse has been of great importance to mankind since the time of conquests and wars. In many battles, victory is attributed to horses and it is said that without these animals it would not have been possible to win wars and conquer new lands, as in the case of the Far West in North America. Horses were used to transport people, tools, weapons and, in some cases, even as a shield against Indian arrows. Nowadays there are several functions for the horse such as sport horses that are used for racing, rodeo, jumping, polo, riding, work, shooting, among others. In events that use sport horses, they often use the teeth as an indicator to calculate their age. The age of the horse is also relevant in the buying and selling of horses, however, most buyers or sellers do not know how to calculate their age. The aim of this project was to produce a manual for estimating the age of horses through their teeth. This manual aims to facilitate the determination of the age of horses as a tool for sporting events, producers, technicians and the general public.

CHAPTER I
EQUINE

Ranking

On the zoological scale the horse belongs to Phylum: vertebrates, Branch: mammals; Class: Ungulates or solipeds; Order: Perissodactyla; Suborder: Hippoide, which at the same time has a single family: Equidae, within which three subfamilies can be distinguished: Hyracoterines, Paleoterines, Equines. a single genus: Equus, which at the same time encloses seven species: ass, Hemicon, Hemipo, Cuaga, Onagro, Zebra and Horse, the latter being the one of interest for this material, the Equus caballus.The horse we know today is very different from its primitive ancestors. Today's horse went through an evolutionary process of approximately 60 million years, moving from the small, no bigger than a fox, cloven-footed Eohippo to the horse we know today. The horse went through major changes, the size being the most obvious, as well as its general conformation and therefore its physiology. Size, conformation of the legs, size of the skull and colour are the most noticeable changes.

Size

The original horse (Eohippus) was no bigger than a fox, so it was not able to support the weight of a man. It then grew to the size of a sheep (Miohippus) and after millions of years, it grew a little more until it was almost the size of a donkey (Pliohippus). It continued to grow during its evolution until it reached Equus fossilis, almost the size of today's horse, which was distributed in America and then became extinct. Subsequently, with the help of man's artificial selection, the horse grew in size until it reached its present size, which on average ranges from 1.50 to 1.80 metres, even more in some breeds.

Foot

One of the most important changes for the horse was the foot, which evolved from the polydactyl of the original horse to the monodactyl of today's horse. The study of the evolution of the foot takes into account the Ehoippus and all its successors up to the Eqqus fossilis. The primitive horse was not only monodactyl but also plantigrade and had five phalanges arranged similarly to the human hand. At this time the horse had a quiet life and was not pursued by predators, so it did not have to walk much.

Later, other animals appeared that forced the horse to flee to protect itself and survive from predators, which meant that when running it had to touch the ground less with its feet in order to move faster, using only one large, thick inner toe instead of five. Therefore, due to this lack of use, the phalanges atrophied until they disappeared, and it is even believed that the fifth phalange in the Eohippo was rudimentary.According to the veterinary anatomists, the mirrors or chestnuts that we can currently observe are the last vestiges of the internal toe, as when dissecting them, we can see that they are innervated and irrigated. In some specimens, there is no presence of these "mirrors" or chestnuts and as they have no physiological function, it is believed that in the future they could disappear completely. Likewise, the horse toe corresponding to the human little finger disappeared due to lack of support on the ground. From Eohippus we then moved on to Orohippus and Mesohippus, characterised by the loss of the inner and outer toes, leaving only three phalanges, represented by the Myohippus. In the same way, the horse's leg evolved into the Equus fossilis. In this way, the horse's support was left with only one toe. This evolution may not have been fully developed, although in today's horses we only see one toe, we still find vestiges of the remaining central toes being represented by the rudimentary metacarpals and metatarsals that are welded to the main toes between 7 and 8 years of age, forming a single bone. It is possible that in the future these phalanges will atrophy and disappear as they have no physiological function. As a consequence of the loss of toes, the horse became more mobile in flexion and extension, making them faster and contributing to the growth in height.

Evolution of Teeth

Another important factor in the evolution of the horse is the teeth.It is now known that the unilateral dental formula of the horse is:(I 3/3 - C 1/1 - PM 3/3 - M 3/3) = 40 teeth. The unilateral dental formula of the primitive horse is:(I 3/3 - C 1/1 - PM 4/4 - M 3/3) = 44 teeth.

I: Incisors C: Canines

PM: Premolars M: Molars

We can clearly observe that there is the presence of one more premolar, however, in the embryo of the current horse there is the presence of the first premolar, commonly called "wolf tooth", which in some cases erupts and disappears when the second premolar molts and the first premolar is no longer replaced. In addition, not only the number of teeth has evolved, but also the shape of the molars, since These pieces, instead of resembling the shape of modern horse teeth, were more similar to the shape of a human being.

Skull

Specialists say that as the horse's toes disappeared until it became monodactyl, the brain also developed and therefore the size of the skull increased until it reached the size of today's horse. It is even believed that in the future the horse's skull may increase even more in size, due to the progressive development of its senses and mental age layers. **Colour**

The colour of the horse's coat was the same for all, a reddish colour, then with time and under the influence of man, a great variety of colours could be acquired, ranging from white to black, passing through all the intermediate colours between these two.

The tail and mane also underwent an evolution, as in primitive horses it was short and coarse haired, whereas in the course of their evolution it grew and straightened until it became long, straight and silky like today's horses, as well as the body hairs which are short and fine in healthy animals.

In summary, the horse has gone through three main stages in its evolution:

1. The original horse was of fox-like size and with a small skull, which stood on five toes and lived on the shores of lakes and swamps. They would correspond to the Eohippus and Orohippus on the new continent and the Palaeothrrium on the old continent.

2. The intermediate horse stage, although it was a little larger in size and had three fingers and the middle finger was the most developed, this preferred to live in dry places and forests. It would correspond to Mesohippus and Miohippus in the new continent and in the old continent it would correspond to Anchitherium and Hipparion.

3. Finally, there is the current type of horse, which is of a larger size, monodactyl,

intelligent, of different colours, with a larger head, developed for speed and adapted to live in any terrain. In the

The new continent would correspond to Pliohippus and Equus fossilis, from which three other types derive, namely Equus caballus robustus or steppe, E. c. pumpeihi or desert, and E. c. nehringi or forest. Of these species, the steppe and forest horses are no longer found in the wild and it is from them that the current horse breeds are derived. Desert horses, on the other hand, still exist in the wild.

Bibliography

Bohorquez, J. I. 1946. The horse: Its origin, evolution and relationship with man. Revista de la Facultad de Medicina Veterinaria y de Zootecnia, 15(90), 48-55.
Durán, R. 2017. The horse manual. Colombia: Grupo Latino Editores. Print.

CHAPTER II
ANATOMY OF THE HEAD OF THE HORSE

** ANATOMICAL PLANES*
**OSTEOLOGY*
**ARTICULATIONS*
** MOUTH CAVITY*

ANATOMICAL PLANES

In order to understand and locate more accurately the direction and parts of the horse's body, some terms are used. For this purpose, it should be known that the plans apply to a quadruped in a natural standing position.

Ventral: It is called ventral to the plane that is directed towards its supporting part, which would be the ground. **Dorsal:** This plane corresponds to the opposite of the ventral plane, i.e. the part of the horse's back.

Medial longitudinal: This plane divides the horse in half into two equal parts. The part closest to this plane is said to be medial or internal and the part furthest from this plane is said to be lateral.

Transverse: This plane cuts the longitudinal plane of the median body perpendicularly in two equal parts. This plane is perpendicular to the mid-sagittal and transverse planes.

Anterior or cranial: This is the end where the head is located.

Posterior or caudal: This is opposite to the anterior or cranial, it is the end where the tail of the animal is located.

Proximal: Refers to being close to the sagittal plane.

Distal: A term used to indicate that it is distant from the sagittal plane.

9

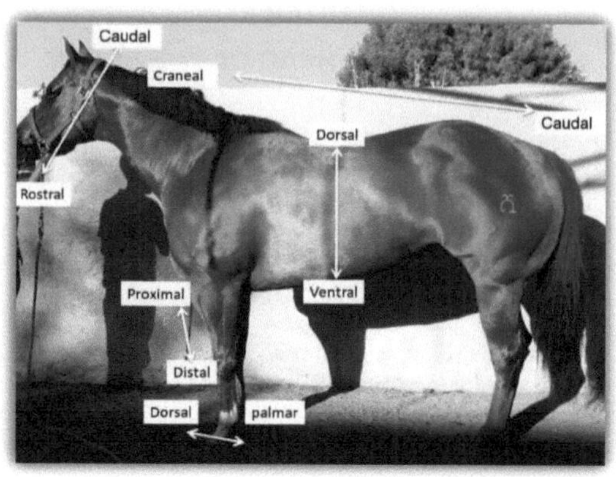

Figure 1. Anatomical drawings.

OSTEOLOGY

Functions of the Bones

The most important functions of bones are to give protection and rigidity to organs. Protection is one of the most vital functions, as in the case of the brain, which is protected by the bones of the skull.

The skeleton of the head is made up of the following bones:

o **Cranial bones:** Occipital, parietal, interparietal, temporal, frontal, ethmoid, sphenoid.

o **Facial bones:** pterygoid, lacrimal, nasal, palatine, concha (turbinate), maxilla, incisors (premaxillary), zygomatic (malar), vomer, mandible, hyoid.

The skull is composed almost entirely of flat bones, which are divided into two surfaces, the inner and outer, of dense bone with a layer of cancellous bone. The occipital, parietal, interparietal, and frontal bones form the posterior and dorsal walls of the skull.

The facial portion can be divided into the orbital, nasal and buccal regions. The orbit is formed by portions of the frontal, lacrimal and zygomatic (malar) bones. In the horse the nasal and buccal portions of the skull are very long.

The airways through the nasal region are bounded dorsally by the nasal bones, laterally by the maxillae and ventrally by the palatine bones.

There are several excavations known as sinuses that are connected to the nasal cavity: the bones where the sinuses are located are the frontal, maxillary, nasal, sphenoid and palatine sinuses.

According to Frandson, the buccal portion carries the maxillae and premaxillae on the roof, the maxillae and premaxillae on the roof. which contain the teeth, as well as the palatine bone. Ventrolaterally, the The mandible completes the buccal portion. The mandible articulates with the temporal bone just in front of the external ear opening. The mandible contains the lower teeth and for similar purposes gives insertion to the muscles of mastication and swallowing.

Occipital bone

The occipital bone is located in the caudal part of the skull, being the base of the head. At its lowest part it is perforated by the foramen magnum, which joins the cranial cavity with the vertebral canal. Above the lateral walls, but without affecting the foramen magnum, is the squamous part. In the lateral proportions they support the occipital condyles which are those that articulate with the atlas. Lateral to the condyle is the cranial surface, which is smooth and concave and contains the jugular process. The ventral condylar fossa is located between the root and the condyle, and along the medial and ventral wall of the condylar fossa is the hypoglossal canal through which the homonymous nerve passes. The ventral surface is circular, while the cranial surface is concave and smooth. It has scaly surfaces where muscles are inserted.

Sphenoids

This bone is located at the base of the skull and the rostral part of the sphenoid sits rostral to the basilar region of the occipital bone. At birth this bone is formed in two distinct parts which are the basisphenoid and the presphenoid.

Basisphenoid bone

This bone consists of a body and two apophyses and two wings. Caudally the body is articulated with the basal portion of the occipital bone and rostrally with the presphenoid; laterally the wings are articulated with the squamosal part of the temporal bone, caudally with the parietal bone and rostrally with the presphenoid. The pterygoid processes articulate medially with the pterygoid bones and rostromedially with the palatine.

Presphenoid bone

This bone is made up of two wings and a body. The body is articulated caudally with the basisphenoid bone and rostrodorsally it articulates with the ethmoid bone, rostroventrally it articulates with the vomer and rostrolaterally with the palatine bone. The wings are articulated dorsolaterally with the frontal bone and caudally with the wings of the basiphoid bone.

Ethmoid Bone

This bone is located rostral to the body and wings of the presphenoid bone, rostrally between the orbits of the frontal bones, and forms part of the formation of the nasal, cranial and paranasal cavity. It is also articulated with the palatine bone, presphenoid and vomer. This bone is made up of four parts; the perpendicular lamina, the cribriform lamina and two labyrinths.

Interparietal Bone

This bone is located centrally in the squamous region of the parietal and occipital bones. It is usually described as a single bone that is ossified to from two lateral cores and often distinctly paired in young foal skulls.

Parietal Bones

These bones make up the bulk of the skull and join together to form the sagittal suture. This bone is articulated with the basisphenoid, temporal, frontal, interparietal and occipital bones. Each has a quadrilateral shape and has four edges and two surfaces; internal surface and external surface. And rostral border, occipital border, interparietal border and squamosal border.

Frontal Bones

These bones are located on the borders of the face and skull, between the nasal bones rostrally and the parietal bones caudally. It is also articulated with the maxillary palatine and squamosal part, presphenoid wing, lacrimal, ethmoid and zygomatic process of the temporal bone. Each is an irregular quadrilateral and consists of an orbital part, a nasal part and a squamosal part.

Temporary Bones

This bone forms the major part of the lateral wall of the skull and is located dorsally the parietal, caudally the occipital, rostrally the frontal and ventrally the basisphenoid. It is also articulated with the hyoid and the mandibular condyle, the zygomatic and the maxilla is articulated with the zygomatic process. In young animals it consists of three parts: petrous, squamosal and tympanic.

Vomer Bone

This is a medial bone that helps the formation of the ventral part of the nasal septum. It is fixed in the sulcus of the palatine process of the maxilla, it is formed by a thin lamina that is folded forming a kind of narrow grooves called sulci. septal plate in which the ventral portion of the perpendicular plate of the ethmoid is housed and the septal cartilage. The uppermost sulcus is articulated with the ethmoid. The caudal part has the presence of lateral wings and pairs that are articulated with the palatine rostrolaterally, caudolaterally with the sphenoid and caudolaterally with the pterygoid.

Maxillae

These bones are the main bones in the upper jaw, and house the molars. They are located in the lateral parts of the face and are articulated with all the facial bones with the temporal and frontal bones. Each can be divided into three apophyses and a body. The lateral facial surface of the body is slightly concave rostrally and convex caudally. In young animals the rostral portion of the surface is convex in the region where the teeth are lodged, as the teeth erupt the face flattens to become concave in older animals. On the caudal side there is a horizontal ridge called the facial crest. In average sized skulls the rostral end of the ridge is located 3 to 4 cm dorsal to the third molar and continues dorsally on the zygomatic bone. Approximately 5 cm dorsal to the rostral end of the ridge is the infraorbital foramen. In the maxillary bone there is a groove rostrodorsally that articulates with the nasal process of the incisor and caudodorsally articulates with the lacrimal and nasal bones.

Incisors

These premaxillary bones form the upper rostral part of the horse and house the incisor teeth. On the opposite side cranially it articulates with the nasal and maxillary bones and the vomer. Each is made up of three apophyses (alveolar, nasal and palatine) and a body. The body in its rostral part is thick, the rostral surface is smooth and convex and is related to the upper lips. The palatal surface there is usually the presence of a foramen slightly caudal to its middle. The alveolar process is thick and curved and has three sockets for the corresponding incisor teeth. The nasal process is located dorsal and caudal to the body and forms a portion of the lateral wall of the nasal cavity. The palatine process is a thin blade and forms the rostral portion of the base of the hard palate.

Palatine Bones

These bones form the caudal portion of the hard palate and are located on each side of the "choanae" (caudal nose). Each of these bones is articulated with bones of the opposite side, frontal, ethmoid, presphenoid, vomer, basisphenoid, pterygoid and maxilla. Each of these bones is slightly twisted in order to form horizontal and perpendicular laminae.

Pterygoid Bones

These bones are thin, curved bony plates that lie on the sides of the choana. It has two surfaces, the medial surface which is thin and forms part of the wall of the choana and the lateral surface which is articulated with the vomer, palatine and basisphenoid bones which together form part of the pterygoid canal.

Nasal Bones

These bones lie rostral to the frontal bones forming the major portion of the roof of the nasal cavity. They are articulated with the opposing frontal bone, lacrimal bone, maxilla and incisors. Caudally it is triangular in shape and broad and rostrally it is pointed.

Tear Bones

These bones lie rostral to the orbit and extend rostrally across the face to the caudal border of the maxilla. This bone articulates dorsally with the nasal and frontal bones, ventrally with the maxilla and zygomatic bone, caudally with the frontal bone and rostrally with the maxilla. The sutures formed are named after the bones of which they are composed.

Zygomatic

These bones lie between the maxilla ventrally and rostrally and the lacrimal dorsally. The temporal process is articulated with the zygomatic process of the temporal bone, each of which is irregularly triangular in outline. The frontal process is absent in the horse.

Jaw

The jaw bone or mandible is the widest bone that makes up the face, these are two halves at birth and after the second or third month they unite to form a single bone. This bone is where the mandibular teeth are located and is articulated by its condylar process with the squamous portion of the temporal bone. It is formed by two vertical branches and a body. The body is a thick, horizontal part which is where the teeth are housed, it is composed of two parts, the molar and the incisor part.

Hyoid bone

This bone is found between the branches of the mandible and its dorsal part is extended somewhat more caudally. It is attached to the styloid process of the petrous region of the temporal bones by pieces of cartilage. It supports the base of the tongue, larynx and pharynx and is made up of several parts; the basohid, the lingual process, the thyroid, the ceratohid, the stylohyoid and the epihyoid.

JOINTS OF THE HEAD

Temporomandibular Joint

This joint is created by the squamous part of the temporal bone on each side and by the branches of the mandible. The articular surfaces differ in size and shape. The squamous portion of the temporal bone is concave-convex and the longitudinal axis leads outwards and slightly rostrally; it is composed of a mandibular orifice which is prolonged by the retroarticular process caudally and a tubercle rostrally. The articular disc is placed between the articulating surface so that it can adapt. The surface is moulded on the temporal and mandibular surface and the circumference is inserted into the articular capsule, thus dividing the articular cavity into two compartments, the inferior and the superior, the latter being the more spacious. The joint capsule is thick and tough and is reinforced by two ligaments. The lateral ligament is obliquely extended and runs across the rostral portion of the lateral surface of the capsule from which it is not allowed to separate. The caudal ligament is an elastic band that inserts ventrally into the line on the caudal aspect of the neck of the mandible and dorsally into the retroarticular process.

Joints and Fibres of the Skull

Most of the bones of the skull are joined to their proximal bones by sutures and only a few by cartilage. There are joints that are made of connective tissue, but there are others that are made of cartilage. Many of these joints become obstructed during development and growth. Generally, these joints are named after the bones that are part of their formation, such as frontonasal, sphenosquamous, etc.

Hyoid Joints

The temporohyoid joint is a slightly mobile joint in which the articular angle of the dorsal end of the stylohyoid bone is inserted by a short cartilage bar into the styloid process of the petrous region of the temporal bone. The arthrohyoid cartilage is between 1 cm and 1.5 cm long. A cartilaginous joint is formed at the junction of the ventral end of the stylohyoid with a dorsal end of the ceratohyoid.

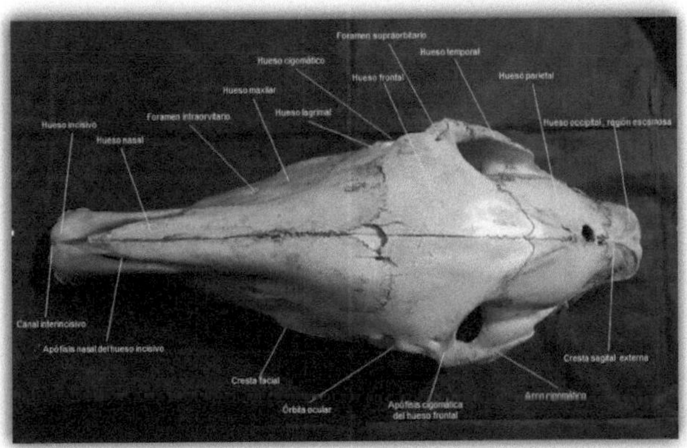

Figure 2. Dorsal view of the skull.

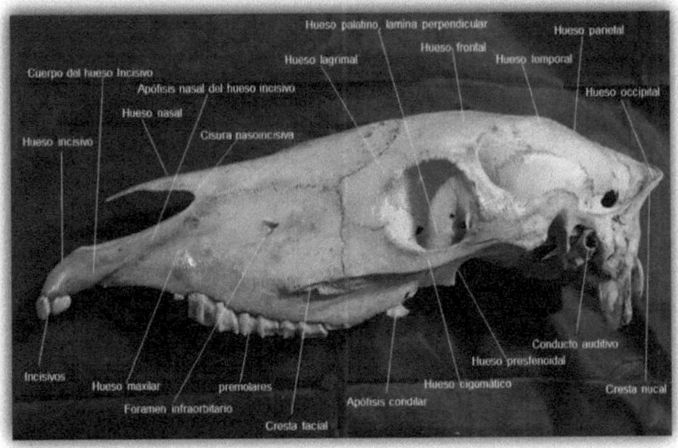

Figure 3. Equine skull left lateral view.

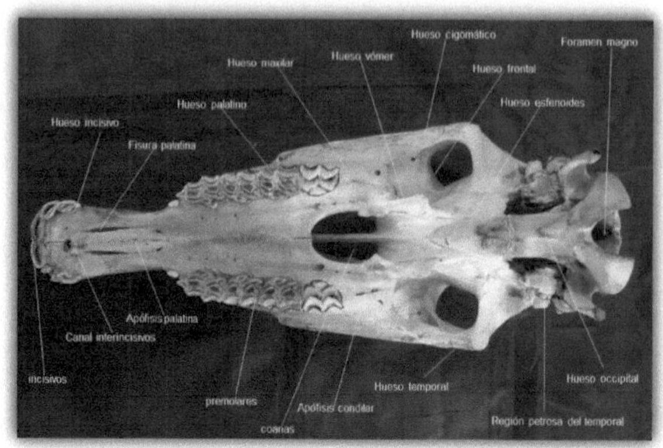

Figure 4. Ventral view of the skull.

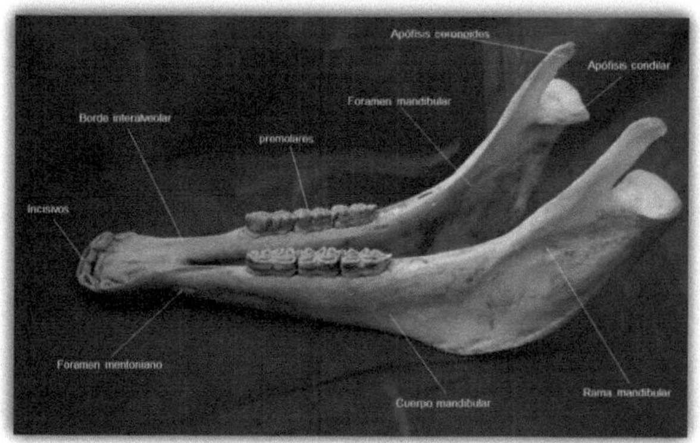

Figure 5. Lower jaw, oblique mid-lateral view.

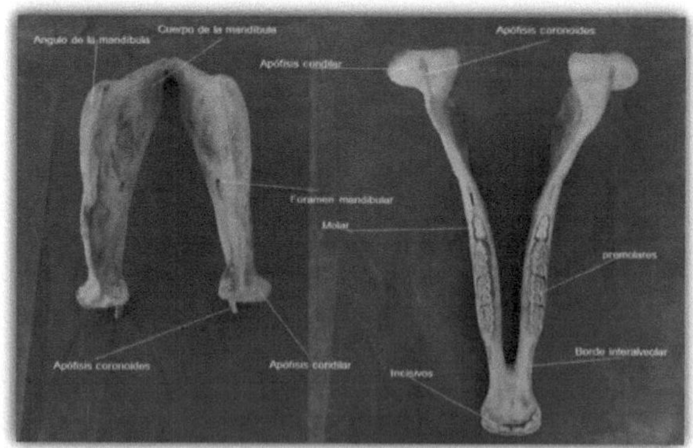

Figure 6. Lower jaw.

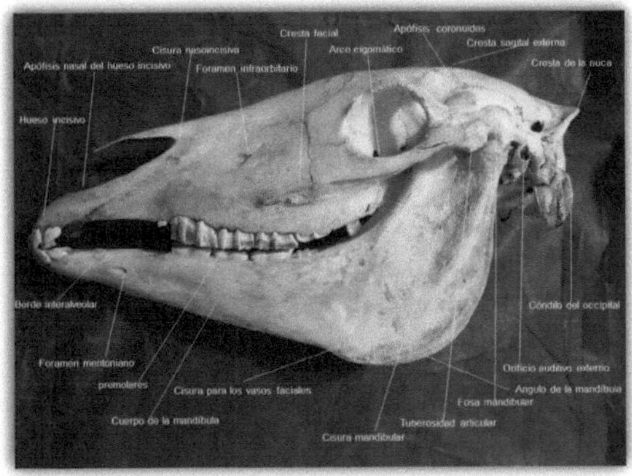

Figure 7. Lateral view of the equine skull and jaw.

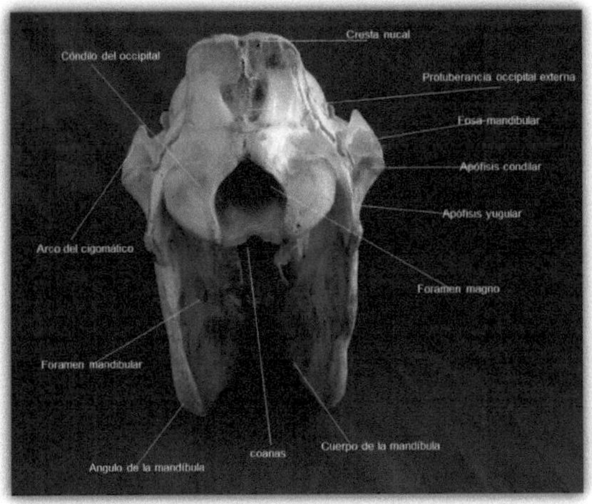

Figure 8. Caudal view of the equine skull and jaw.

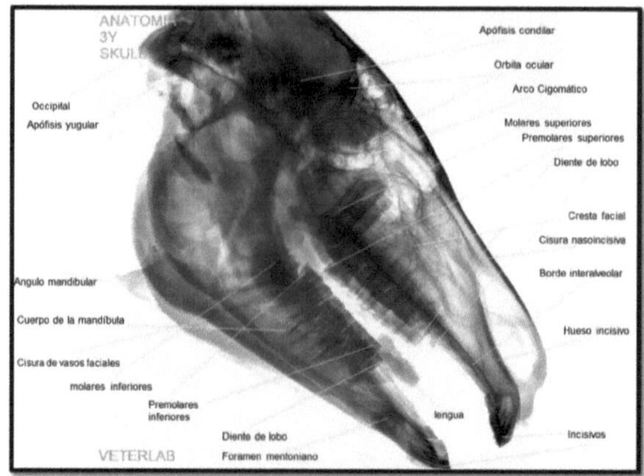

Figure 9. Left lateral radiograph of a three-year-old equine.

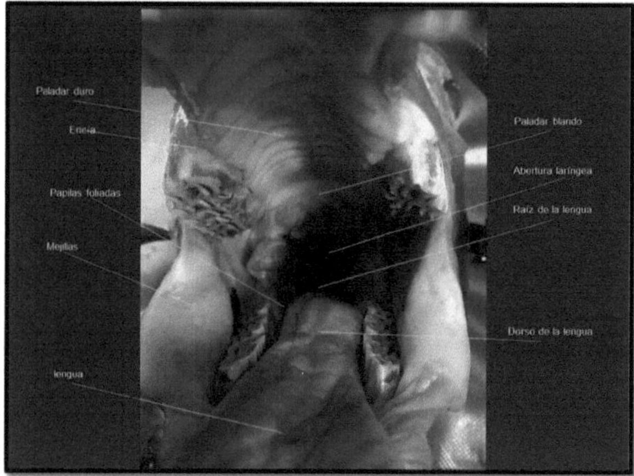

Figure 10. Internal view of the mouth.

Bibliography

Frandson, R. D., and Spurgeon, T. L. 1995. Anatomy and physiology of domestic animals. Interamericana/McGraw-Hill.

Sisson, S., and Grossman, J. D. 2003. Anatomy of domestic animals . Barcelona: Masson .

CHAPTER III

NUTRITION

FUELING
**SHAPES*
**GRANOS*
**NUTRITIONAL REQUIREMENTS*

Feeding

The horse is a herbivorous animal without a rumen, but has a microbial fermentation in the hindgut exactly in the caecum and colon, so the horse can consume fibrous food. There are microorganisms in the equine intestine very similar to those of ruminants, mainly bacteria, protozoa and fungl. There Is a fermentation in the caecum which results in the production of carbon dioxide, volatile fatty acids, mainly acetate, propionate and butyrate. Methane is also produced, but in small quantities, approximately less than 3 % of the amount of feed ingested. Volatile fatty acids are very easily absorbed in the hindgut and are used as a source of energy. It is said that 30 % or more of the energy used by the horse comes from these volatile fatty acids. Propionate can also be an important source of glucose production, however, acetate and butyrate are not gluconeogenic. The horse does not utilise fibre from feed as efficiently as ruminants because the microflora of the hindgut do not have as much time to ferment the feed as ruminants and therefore the equine digestion is faster. The hindgut bacteria also produce vitamins and water-soluble proteins which are not utilised in large quantities, as the hindgut does not absorb them well. The horse is mainly fed on forage or forage-equivalent feed and must consume more than 1 % dry matter of its live weight. We must be aware that when we feed a horse we are not only feeding the horse, but also the micro-organisms in the digestive tract. Therefore, proper nutrition helps with the reduction of cases of digestive problems such as colic and others. It is preferable to give more feed repetitions to the horse, especially if the diet is very rich in energy and poor in roughage, we should offer at least 3 meals to

21

avoid affecting the microbial activity and the liquid in the intestine and thus avoid digestive disorders.

Forages

Forages are those plants or herbaceous plants that are in the soil and are used to feed some herbivorous animals, such as horses. There are different types of fodder production, the most important of which are hay and silage. Forage supports normal microbial activity in the digestive tract and provides nutrients such as vitamins, minerals, energy and protein. Grass or legume forages can be offered. It is important to consider the nutritional content and cost of the feed offered to horses, including its palatability to the animal. The condition of the fodder, i.e. free from moulds and fungi that can affect it, should also be considered. Leguminous forages usually have a higher percentage of protein and are widely used in lactating mares and weaned foals due to their high protein requirement.

Grains

Oats are one of the main grains used in horse feed because of their palatability and safety. In addition, oats are higher in protein and lower in energy than other grains, and can be offered whole or crumbled. Crumbled oats increase the dry matter digestibility by 5 to 7 %, and are recommended for feeding to young foals and older horses that have problems with their teeth. On the other hand, corn is an excellent source of energy, providing about twice as much energy as oats, and corn is a very economical ingredient.

Table 1. Daily nutrient requirements of the mature 200 kg horse.

	weight	GDP/Milk	ED	PC	Lys	Ca	P
Type	kg	kg/day	Mcal	g	G	g	G
Jobless adult							
Minimum	200		6.1	216	9.3	8.0	5.6
Average	200		6.7	252	10.8	8.0	5.6
Elevated	200		7.3	288	12.4	8.0	5.6
Work							
Light exercise	200		8.0	280	12.0	12.0	7.2
Moderate exercise	200		9.3	307	13.2	14.0	8.4
Heavy exercise	200		10.7	345	14.8	16.0	11.6
Very heavy exercise	200		13.8	345	17.3	16.0	11.6
Stallions							
Non-breeding	200		7.3	288	12.4	8.0	5.6
Breeding	200		8.7	316	13.6	12.0	7.2
Pregnant mares							
Less than 5 months	200		6.7	252	10.8	8.0	5.6
5 months	201	0.05	6.8	274	11.8	8.0	5.6
6 months	203	0.07	7.0	282	12.1	8.0	5.6
7 months	206	0.10	7.2	291	12.5	11.2	8.0
8 months	209	0.13	7.4	304	13.1	11.2	8.0
9 months	214	0.16	7.7	319	13.7	14.4	10.5
10 months	219	0.21	8.1	336	14.5	14.4	10.5
11 months	226	0.26	8.6	357	15.4	14.4	10.5
Lactating mares							
1 month	200	6.52	12.7	614	33.9	23.6	15.3
2 months	200	6.48	12.7	612	33.8	23.6	15.2
3 months	200	5.98	12.2	587	32.1	22.4	14.4
4 months	200	5.42	11.8	559	30.3	16.7	10.5
5 months	200	4.88	11.3	532	28.5	15.8	9.9
6 months	200	4.36	10.9	506	26.8	15.0	9.3
Growth							
4 months	67	0.34	5.3	268	11.5	15.6	8.7
6 months	86	0.29	6.2	270	11.6	15.5	8.6
12 months	128	0.18	7.5	338	14.5	15.1	8.4
18 months	155	0.11	7.7	320	13.7	14.8	8.2
24 months	172	0.07	7.5	308	13.2	14.7	8.1

(NRC, 2012).

Table 2. Daily nutrient requirements of the 400 kg mature horse.

Type	weight	GDP/Milk	ED	PC	Lys	Ca	P
	kg	kg/day	Mcal	g	g	g	g
Jobless adult							
Minimum	400		12.1	432	18.6	16.0	11.2
Average	400		13.3	504	21.7	16.0	11.2
Elevated	400		14.5	576	24.8	16.0	11.2
Work							
Light exercise	400		16.0	559	24.1	24.0	14.4
Moderate exercise	400		18.6	614	26.4	28.0	16.8
Heavy exercise	400		21.3	689	29.6	32.0	23.2
Very heavy exercise	400		27.6	804	34.6	32.0	23.2
Stallions							
Non-breeding	400		14.5	576	24.8	16.0	11.2
Breeding	400		17.4	631	27.1	24.0	14.4
Pregnant mares							
Less than 5 months	400		13.3	504	21.7	16.0	11.2
5 months	403	0.11	13.7	548	23.6	16.0	11.2
6 months	407	0.15	13.9	563	24.2	16.0	11.2
7 months	412	0.19	14.3	583	25.1	22.4	16.0
8 months	419	0.26	14.8	607	26.1	22.4	16.0
9 months	427	0.33	15.4	637	27.4	28.8	21.0
10 months	439	0.42	16.2	673	28.9	28.8	21.0
11 months	453	0.52	17.1	714	30.7	28.8	21.0
Lactating mares							
1 month	400	13.04	25.4	1228	67.8	47.3	30.6
2 months	400	12.96	25.3	1224	67.5	47.1	30.5
3 months	400	11.96	24.5	1174	64.2	44.7	28.8
4 months	400	10.84	23.6	1118	60.5	33.3	20.9
5 months	400	9.76	22.7	1064	57.0	31.6	19.7
6 months	400	8.72	21.8	1012	53.5	30.0	18.6
Growth							
4 months	135	0.67	10.6	535	23.0	31.3	17.4
6 months	173	0.58	12.4	541	23.3	30.9	17.2
12 months	257	0.36	15.0	677	29.1	30.1	16.7
18 months	310	0.23	15.4	639	27.5	29.6	16.5
24 months	343	0.14	15.0	616	26.5	29.3	16.3

(NRC, 2012).

Table 3. Daily nutrient requirements of the 500 kg mature horse.

Type	weight kg	GDP/Milk kg/day	ED Mcal	PC g	Lys g	Ca g	P G
Jobless adult							
Minimum	500		15.2	540	23.2	20.0	14.0
Average	500		16.7	630	27.1	20.0	14.0
Elevated	500		18.2	720	31.0	20.0	14.0
Work							
Light exercise	500		20.0	699	30.1	30.0	18.0
Moderate exercise	500		23.3	768	33.0	35.0	21.0
Heavy exercise	500		26.6	862	37.1	40.0	29.0
Very heavy exercise	500		34.5	1004	43.2	40.0	29.0
Stallions							
Non-breeding	500		18.2	720	31.0	20.0	14.0
Breeding	500		21.8	789	33.9	30.0	18.0
Pregnant mares							
Less than 5 months	500		16.7	630	27.1	20.0	14.0
5 months	504	0.14	17.1	685	29.5	20.0	14.0
6 months	508	0.18	17.4	704	30.3	20.0	14.0
7 months	515	0.24	17.9	729	31.3	28.0	20.0
8 months	523	0.32	18.5	759	32.7	28.0	20.0
9 months	534	0.41	19.2	797	34.3	36.0	26.3
10 months	548	0.52	20.2	841	36.2	36.0	26.3
11 months	566	0.65	21.4	893	38.4	36.0	26.3
Lactating mares							
1 month	500	16.30	31.7	1535	84.8	59.1	38.3
2 months	500	16.20	31.7	1530	84.4	58.9	38.1
3 months	500	14.95	30.6	1468	80.3	55.9	36.0
4 months	500	13.55	29.4	1398	75.7	41.7	26.2
5 months	500	12.20	28.3	1330	71.2	39.5	24.7
6 months	500	10.90	27.2	1265	66.9	37.4	23.2
Growth							
4 months	168	0.84	13.3	669	28.8	39.1	21.7
6 months	216	0.72	15.5	676	29.1	38.6	21.5
12 months	321	0.45	18.8	846	36.4	37.7	20.9
18 months	387	0.29	19.2	799	34.4	37.0	20.6
24 months	429	0.18	18.7	770	33.1	36.7	20.4

(NRC, 2012).

Table 4. Daily nutrient requirements of the 600 kg mature horse.

Type	weight	GDP/Milk	ED	PC	Lys	Ca	P
	kg	kg/day	Mcal	g	g	g	g
Jobless adult							
Minimum	600		18.2	648	27.9	24.0	16.8
Average	600		20.0	756	32.5	24.0	16.8
Elevated	600		21.8	864	37.2	24.0	16.8
Work							
Light exercise	600		24.0	839	36.1	36.0	21.6
Moderate exercise	600		28.0	921	39.6	42.0	25.2
Heavy exercise	600		32.0	1034	44.5	48.0	34.8
Very heavy exercise	600		41.4	1205	51.8	48.0	34.8
Stallions							
Non-breeding	600		21.8	864	37.2	24.0	16.8
Breeding	600		26.1	947	40.7	36.0	21.6
Pregnant mares							
Less than 5 months	600		20.0	756	32.5	24.0	16.8
5 months	604	0.16	20.5	822	35.3	24.0	16.8
6 months	610	0.22	20.9	845	36.3	24.0	16.8
7 months	618	0.29	21.5	874	37.6	33.6	24.0
8 months	628	0.38	22.2	911	39.2	33.6	24.0
9 months	641	0.49	23.1	956	41.1	43.2	31.5
10 months	658	0.63	24.2	1009	43.4	43.2	31.5
11 months	679	0.78	25.7	1072	46.1	43.2	31.5
Lactating mares							
1 month	600	19.56	38.1	1842	101.7	70.9	45.9
2 months	600	19.44	38.0	1836	101.3	70.7	45.7
3 months	600	17.94	36.7	1761	96.4	67.1	43.2
4 months	600	16.26	35.3	1677	90.8	50.0	31.4
5 months	600	14.64	34.0	1596	85.5	47.4	29.6
6 months	600	13.08	32.7	1518	80.3	44.9	27.9
Growth							
4 months	202	1.01	15.9	803	34.5	46.9	26.1
6 months	259	0.87	18.6	811	34.9	46.4	25.8
12 months	385	0.54	22.5	1015	43.6	45.2	25.1
18 months	465	0.34	23.1	959	41.2	44.5	24.7
24 months	515	0.22	22.4	924	39.7	44.0	24.4

(NRC, 2012).

Table 5. Daily nutrient requirements of the 900 kg mature horse.

Type	weight kg	GDP/Milk kg/day	ED Mcal	PC g	Lys g	Ca g	P g
Jobless adult							
Minimum	900		27.3	972	41.8	36.0	25.2
Average	900		30.0	1134	48.8	36.0	25.2
Elevated	900		32.7	1296	55.7	36.0	25.2
Work							
Light exercise	900		36.0	1259	54.1	54.0	32.4
Moderate exercise	900		42.0	1382	59.4	63.0	37.8
Heavy exercise	900		48.0	1551	66.7	72.0	52.2
Very heavy exercise	900		62.1	1808	77.7	72.0	52.2
Stallions							
Non-breeding	900		32.7	1296	55.7	36.0	25.2
Breeding	900		39.2	1421	61.1	54.0	32.4
Pregnant mares							
Less than 5 months	900		30.0	1134	48.8	36.0	25.2
5 months	906	0.24	30.8	1233	53.0	36.0	25.2
6 months	915	0.33	31.4	1267	54.5	36.0	25.2
7 months	927	0.44	32.2	1311	56.4	50.4	36.0
8 months	942	0.57	33.3	1367	58.8	50.4	36.0
9 months	962	0.74	34.6	1434	61.7	64.8	47.3
10 months	987	0.94	36.4	1514	65.1	64.8	47.3
11 months	1019	1.17	38.5	1607	69.1	64.8	47.3
Lactating mares							
1 month	900	29.34	54.4	2763	152.6	106.4	68.9
2 months	900	29.16	54.3	2754	152.0	106.0	68.6
3 months	900	26.91	52.4	2642	144.5	100.6	64.9
4 months	900	24.39	50.3	2516	136.2	75.0	47.1
5 months	900	21.96	48.3	2394	128.2	71.1	44.4
6 months	900	19.62	46.3	2277	120.5	67.4	41.8
Growth							
4 months	303	1.52	23.9	1204	51.8	70.3	39.1
6 months	389	1.30	28.0	1217	52.3	69.5	38.7
12 months	578	0.82	33.8	1522	65.5	67.8	37.7
18 months	697	0.51	34.6	1438	61.8	66.7	37.1
24 months	773	0.32	33.7	1386	59.6	66.0	36.7

(NRC, 2012).

Bibliography

Church, D., Pond, W., & Pond, K. 2017. Fundamentals of Animal Nutrition and Feeding. Mexico : Limusa.

N.R.C. 1989. Nutrient requirements of horses. Fifth revised edition. Washington: National Academy Press.

N.R.C. 2012. Nutrient requirements of horses. Sixth revised edition. Washington D.C: Library of congress catalogin-in-publication data .

*COMPOSITION
*DENTAL NOMENCLATURE
*DENTAL FORMULAS
*MORPHOLOGY
*TYPES OF TEETH

Composition

The teeth are hard papillary structures that are attached to the upper and lower jaws, they are mainly organs of pressure and mastication, although they are also a defence tool The tooth is divided into three parts which are the crown, the neck and the root. The crown is that part that protrudes from the gum (clinical crown) or that part that is covered by enamel (dental crown) and has a cylindrical or triangular shape. The neck is the portion that joins the crown to the root, the latter being the part of the tooth that is embedded in the mandibular alveolus, which at its lower extremity has an opening through which nerves, veins and arteries pass, called the apical foramen or apex. The tooth is made up of soft and hard substances. The soft substances include the dental pulp and the periodontium, and the hard substances include the enamel, cementum and dentine or ivory.

The enamel

It is a more superficial layer of varying thickness that surrounds and covers the dentine and shapes the outside of the dental crown. It is the hardest tissue in the body. It is distinguished mainly by its whiteness and density and cleanliness. Its colour can vary from bluish white to dull yellow. Its hardness is due to its high level of phosphate and calcium fluoride minerals. It is the most mineralised structure in the body and has only 2 to 8 % organic matter, and in calcination studies it has been found that half of this percentage is moisture. Enamel is the first to finish calcifying before other dental tissues. The enamel is formed by cylindrical and parallel vertices that go from the line that delimits the dentine with the enamel to the superficial part of the crown. These prisms when viewed under a microscope with a cross-section are usually circular or hexagonal in shape and their composition is an apatite or fluorapatite.

Cement

It is a compact bone-like substance, the outermost covering of the root, which forms an embedded layer over the dentine of the roots of all teeth.

Dentine

It is a hard, yellowish-white bone tissue produced by odontoblasts, also known as ground substance, as it is the main part of the tooth that runs from the root to the crown, covering the surface of the dental pulp. It can be distinguished from bone as it is richer in minerals and has a lower presence of organic matter and calcium carbonate and contains up to 70 percent apatite (mineral salts).

The dental pulp

It is a kind of papilla that emerges from the bottom of the alveolus, which is lodged in the internal turbinate and is formed by connective tissue rich in nerves and blood vessels.The periodontium is a fibrous membrane whose function is the junction between the wall of the alveolus and the external surface of the root. The following results were obtained by calcination analysis of the tissues.

Table 6. Chemical composition of the tooth.

	Enamel	Dentine	Cement
Water	2.3 %	13.5 %	32.0 %
Organic matter	1.7 %	17.5 %	22.0 %
Ashes	96.0 %	69.0 %	46.0 %

Dental nomenclature

Unlike human dental nomenclature, equine dental nomenclature is guided by the modified triad system which uses three digits to locate each tooth numbered in four quadrants in a clockwise direction starting with 101 which corresponds to the first upper right incisor and ending with 411 which corresponds to the third lower right molar. There is another type of nomenclature such as the traditional system where it is numbered by dental group using the first letter and the part number e.g. I 1, C1, P2, M3.

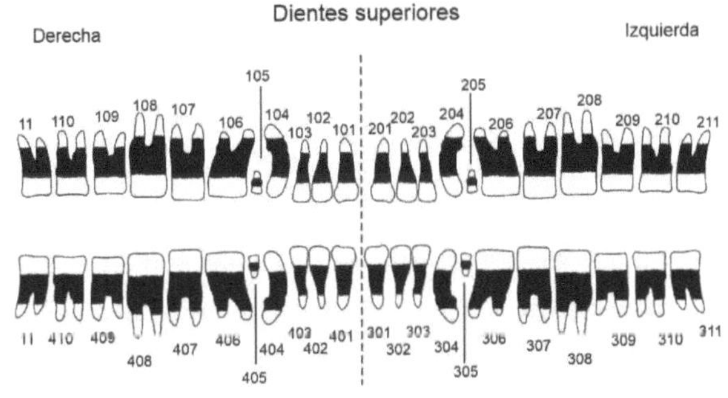

Figure 11. Modified triad system.

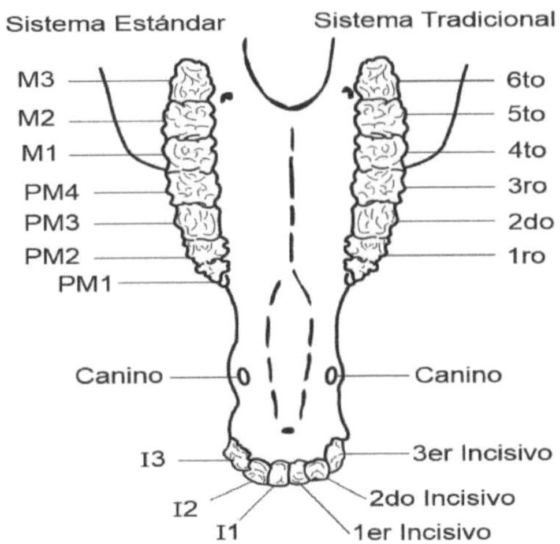

Figure 12. Equine dental nomenclature.

Dental Formulas

When we talk about dental formula we refer to the way of expressing the number of teeth that an animal has, in the form of broken numbers indicating in the upper part the number of each type of tooth in the jaw and, in the lower fraction, the number of teeth that the jaw has, but only of half of the mouth. In other words, to know the total number of teeth an animal has, it is necessary to multiply the data by two. This formula varies according to age, it is unequal for primary and permanent teeth. The equine dental formula is age and sex related and is as follows: First dentition corresponding to deciduous teeth: 2(I 3/3, C 0/0, PM 3/3) = 24 dental weights for both sexes.In the second dentition, which are the permanent teeth, the number of teeth varies according to sex: Males: 2(I 3/3, C 1/1, PM 3-4/3-4, M 3/3) = 40-44 teeth Females: 2(I 3/3, C 0/0, PM 3-4/3-4, M 3/3) = 36-44 teeth. The difference in the number of teeth between males and females corresponds to the fact that in females the canines are generally absent, however, they may appear in some cases. The variability in the number of teeth in the premolars for both sexes corresponds to the presence or absence of the first premolar, also known as the "wolf tooth". This tooth can be present in both the upper and lower arches, although it is more likely to be present in the upper arch, being smaller than the others and with shorter roots.

Morphology

All teeth are morphologically different, however they have characteristics that are compatible for all teeth. Each tooth is divided into three parts for study: root, neck and crown. To better locate the faces of the teeth we must divide the mouth with an imaginary line into two sides, left and right. If we compare the dental piece with a cube we can see that it has 6 faces of which two are perpendicular to its own axis and 4 faces are parallel to its own axis which are called axial. Of the two remaining faces that are perpendicular to the axis, one is called the occlusal or masticatory face and the other is the cervical plane that joins the root to the crown at the neck.

Axial faces

They are called axial faces because they are parallel to the longitudinal axis of the tooth. There are four axial faces, two of which contact or are in close proximity to the teeth.

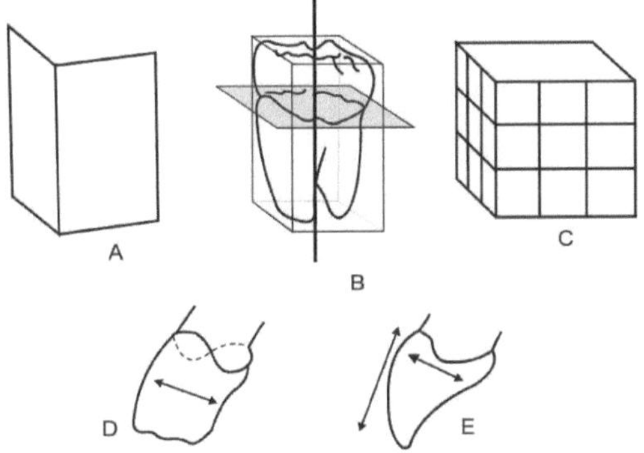

Figure 13. Representation of axial faces.

Mesial Face

This face is the one that is closest or closest to the median plane of the head (from the Greek meso, in the middle).

Distal Face

This is the face that is furthest away or distant from the median plane of the head. The other two remaining faces are called free faces because they do not make contact with any other anatomical structure and when they do make contact with the tongue, lips or cheeks this contact can be interrupted.

Vestibular Face

The vestibular side of the tooth that is in contact with the lateral vestibule of the oral cavity is called the vestibular side in posterior teeth, and the side that is in contact with the lips is called the labial side in anterior teeth.

Lingual Face

The lingual side is the name given to all that part of the tooth that is in contact with the tongue, both in the front teeth and in the back, upper and lower teeth. In the upper teeth, although they are further away from the tongue, they can make contact with the tongue.

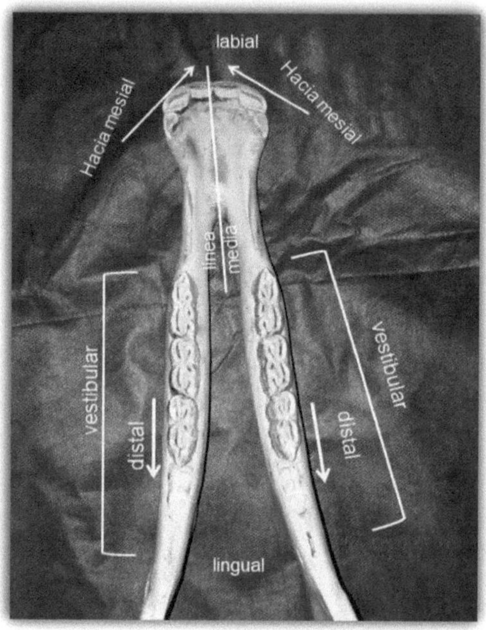

Figure 14. Axial faces.

Types of teeth

Horses' teeth are classified as heterodont because they have different types of teeth such as incisors, canines, premolars and molars. They are also classified as diphyodont because they have two types of teeth, the temporary or milk teeth and the permanent or cement dentition. In the first weeks of life the first milk teeth appear, which will later be replaced by the permanent teeth that will accompany the animal throughout its life. The teeth of horses are divided into four different groups depending on their shape, position and function: incisors, canines, premolars and molars.

Incisors

They are located in front and embedded in the premaxilla and in the mandible, forming a semicircle between the 6 incisors. Their main function is to cut grass. In its crown there is a cavity or invagination covered with enamel and cementum with a depth of more than one centimetre known as the infundibulum or corneum. As the tooth wears down, a central ring of enamel appears apart from the peripheral enamel. This cavity becomes darker due to the food that is deposited in it, and is known as a mark or cup. The opening of the infundibulum is large and rounded in its deepest part and progressively decreases in size, sloping towards the lingual part of the tooth. The distal part of the pulp cavity passes through the lingual side of the infundibulum, which is why, as the tooth wears down, the pulp cavity that was closed by a layer of dentine appears on the occlusal part known as the dental star before the infundibulum disappears completely. Each tooth wears evenly from the crown to its apex and curves longitudinally. The root is the apical part and a part of it can be called a reserve crown because it advances from the alveolus. When the incisors start to The occlusal surfaces are approximately 7 cm long and the occlusal surface is larger mediolaterally than rostrocaudally. The upper incisors are wider and more convex than the lower teeth. The labial or vestibular surfaces are flatter transversely than the lingual surface. The upper incisors at the ends are wider than the lower incisors. On the labial surface of the upper incisor there is a longitudinal groove that starts halfway from the occlusal surface towards the apex and continues approximately three quarters of the way from the apex if measured on an unworn tooth. The crown is covered by the gum, which is why it is smaller in corpses or living animals than in a skull. Part of the apical end of the tooth is open at the beginning and gradually closes because dentine and cementum adhere to it, except for a small foramen through which vessels and nerves pass. The occlusal shape of the tooth as it wears down changes from an oval shape, then a circular shape and finally a triangular to rectangular shape. The upper and lower incisors erupt at the same time. The change of shape of the infundibulum, the appearance of the dental star and the disappearance of the infundibulum usually occurs from the first incisor to the third incisor, but in some cases it may disappear first in the extreme incisor before the other two. The infundibulum of the upper teeth is deeper than that of the lower teeth and the infundibulum of the lower teeth disappears later. The incisors more proximal to the medial plane are called pincers or blades, immediately distal to these are called middle or median and the most distal are called wedges or end teeth. The longitudinal sulcus of the vestibular part of the upper incisor generally makes presence at 10 years of age of the end of the gum towards the occlusal part of the tooth reached the occlusal side at about 20 years of age. Then the sulcus on the gum side begins to disappear until it disappears completely on the occlusal side of the incisor at the age of 30.The dental star appears at the age of 8 years on the first incisor and later on the other incisors. At first the dental star appears in the occlusal part of the incisor on the side rostral to the infundibulum and as the infundibulum becomes small and circular the dental star grows until the infundibulum disappears and only the dental star remains in the occlusal part of the incisor. In order to differentiate between primary teeth and permanent teeth, it is necessary to know that primary teeth are whiter, longer than wide, smaller, the occlusal surface is more oval, they are smooth without grooves on the labial side, their neck is well defined and marked at the insertion with the gum and the infundibulum is shallower. The permanent teeth are more yellow to brown stained, larger, longer than wide, rectangular in shape and have grooves on the labial surface.

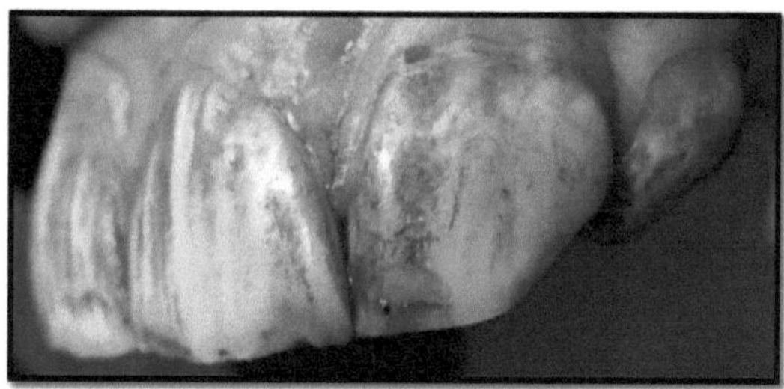

(a)

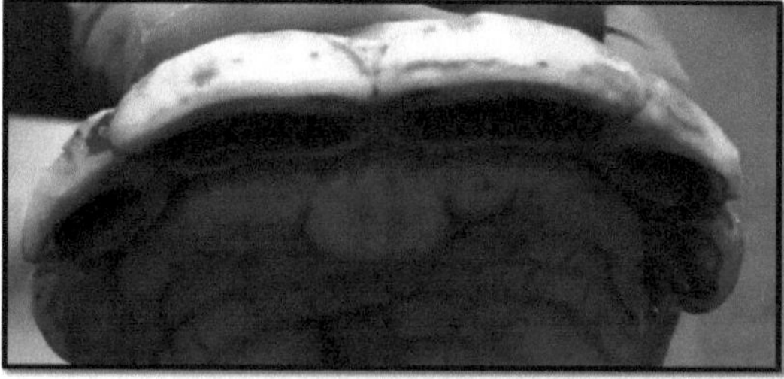

(b)

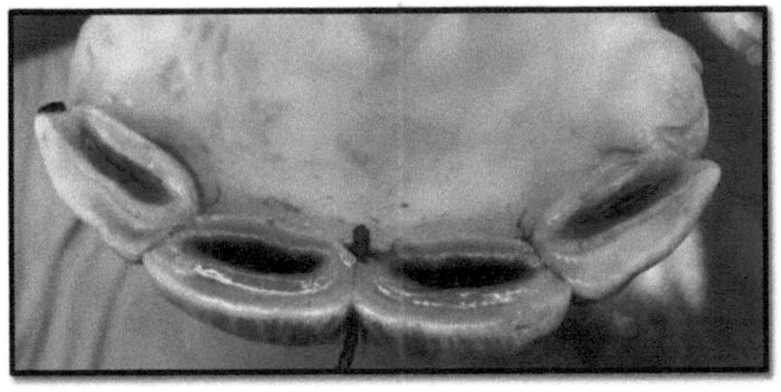

(c)

Figure 15. Incisors (a) labial, (b) palatal and (c) ventral.

Canines

The canines are located after the incisors from vestibular to cranial and their main function is to tear food. They are only present in the permanent dentition. The diastema or bar is the interdental space between the canines and premolars and this is larger when there is an absence of canines. Canines are usually only present in males and are absent in mares. The upper canine is located at an intermediate point rostrally between the last incisor and the first premolars and divides the diastema between incisors and premolars. However, the lower canines are located closer to the last incisor. The upper canines usually never make contact with the lower canines when the mouth is closed, although there is wear and tear from food. They are small and simple teeth with no infundibulum and have a long pulp cavity and an open root. This tooth curves slightly from the alveolus with age.

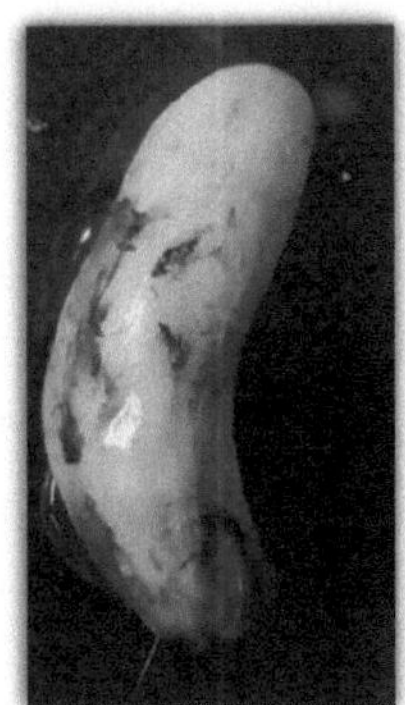

Figure 16. Canine tooth.

37

Premolars and molars

The premolars and molars are located at the end after the canines with the premolars appearing first and the molars are the last and only appear in the cement dentition. Their function is to crush and grind the food. The first premolar, also called "dens lupinus" is commonly absent and when present it is a very small tooth. The other premolars and molars are very similar to each other, they are large and quadrangular in shape with the exception of the second premolar and the last molar which has only three sides. Each molar has 2 deep infundibulae. A large part of the crown is submerged in the alveolus and as the tooth advances from the alveolus there is a functional crown of approximately 2 cm. At the apex of the crown are the roots, which close with time due to the adhesion of dentine and cementum, so that when the horse is 14 years old they are almost closed except for the apical foramen. The occlusal part of these teeth are molariform and have a lophodontic configuration. The caudal part in the third molar is more compressed. On the buccal surface of each upper molar there is the presence of two wide longitudinal grooves which are separated from each other by a narrow protruding ridge. Each upper piece is slightly more inclined towards the buccal side where the crown is more visible. The molars laterally have two roots and a thick root on the medial side which tends to be double. Premolar 2 is the shortest of the molars, followed by molar 1.

The lower molars and premolars form a straight mandibular line and are inclined on their occlusal side to the opposite side than the upper teeth, i.e. they are slightly inclined to the lingual side. The space between the left and right line is smaller in the lower teeth than in the upper teeth. The occlusal surface of the lower molars is in contact with the lingual side of the occlusal surface of the upper molars. In the upper molars there are five divisions of the pulp cavity, so that on the occlusal side of the teeth there are five dental stars, each star is a slightly worn beak on the lower side. The inner and outer enamel is harder than the dentine, so the enamel wears more slowly. The infundibulum is initially incomplete at the lingual edge of the occlusal part and becomes more complete as it wears. The pulp cavity of the lower molars has two main divisions and several secondary diverticula, each of which corresponds to a dental star. Three lingual diverticula are present. Each pulp cavity has an additional lingual diverticulum in the caudal and rostral part of the tooth. On the other side of the upper molars, the buccal cusps are called paracones and metacones and the lingual cusps are called protoconules, protocones and hypocones. The lingual cusps of the lower molars are called protoconulids, metaconoids, metastyles, entoconulids and hypoconulids and the buccal side cusps are called protoconoids and hypoconoids. In the second premolar the protoconulids and in the third molar the hypoconulids are larger because these molars are the end of the dental series.

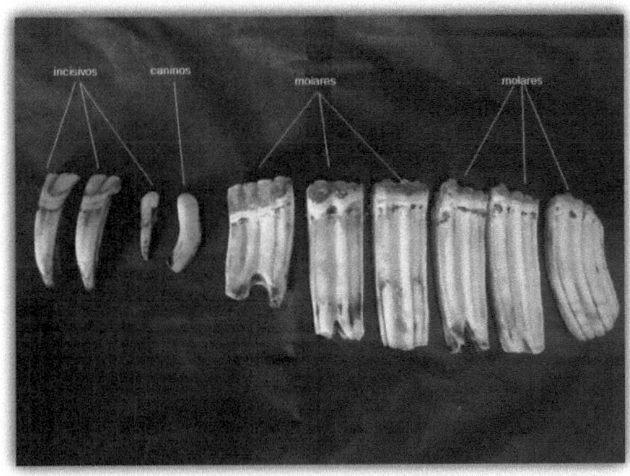

Figure 17. Lower teeth.

CHAPTER V
AGE ESTIMATION

This chapter shows pictures and descriptive information about age identification in equines by looking at their teeth. You will find clear pictures with a description explaining each image so that you can better understand it and determine the age of a horse.

Table 7. Estimation of equine age.

First stage: 15 days	
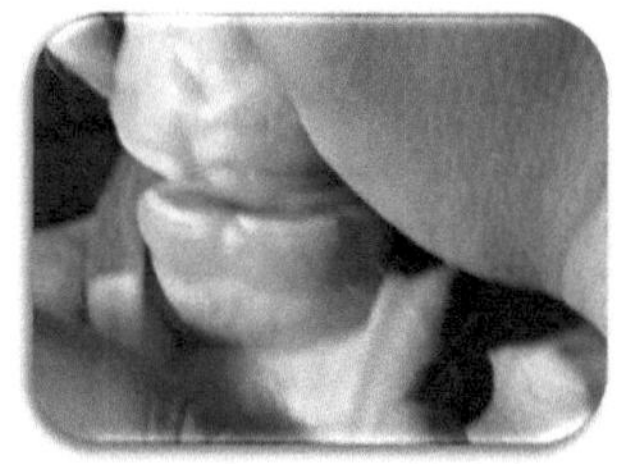	The first primary incisors begin to appear at 15 days of age.
Second phase: 6 months	
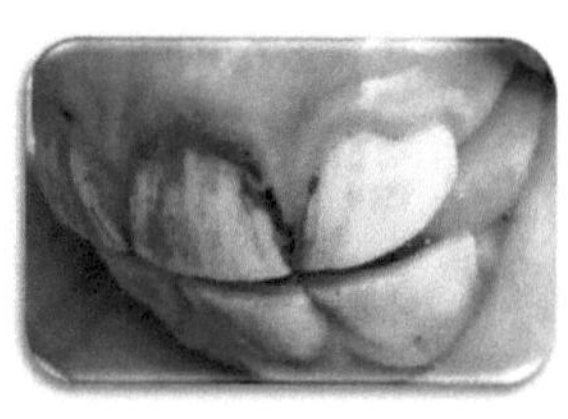	Presence of: -First primary incisor: present and growing. -Second temporary incisor: present and growing. -Third primary incisor: no At this stage of 6 months of age, the first and second milk incisors are present. third incisors still absent.
Third stage of (12 months): 1 year	
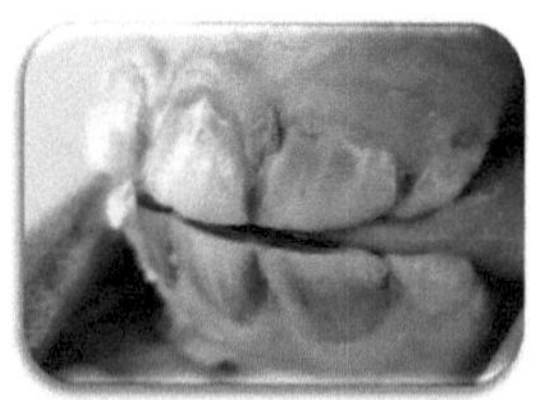	Presence of: -First temporary incisor: present reaching the rachis. -Second temporary incisor: present and growing. -Third primary incisor: present and growing. At this stage of one year, the first incisors are present and reaching the raking stage, while the second and third incisors are also growing.
Stage four (18 months): 1.5 years	

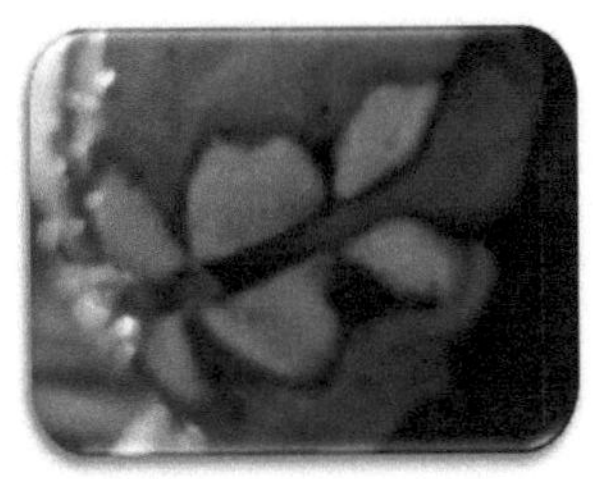

	Presence of: -First primary incisor: present reaching shaving -Second temporary incisor: present reaching shaving -Third primary incisor: present during growth At this stage of 18 months of age the first and second milk incisors are present and reaching shaving, while the third milk incisors are growing.

Fifth stage of (24 months): 2 years

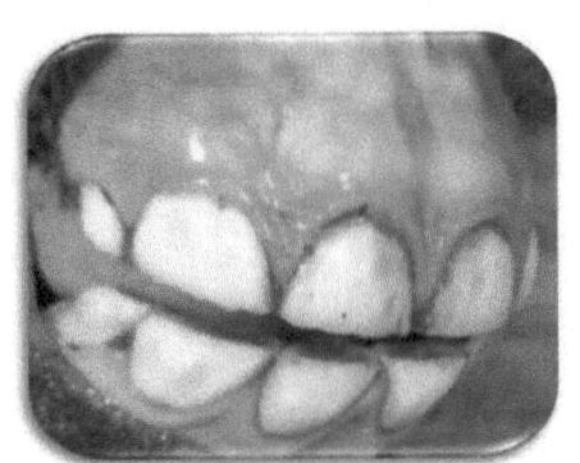

	Presence of: -First temporary incisor: present and reaching shaving. -Second temporary incisor: present and reaching shaving. -Third incisor: present and reaching shaving. At this stage, at the age of two years we can find the first, second and third primary incisors present and reaching their shaving.

Sixth stage (30 months): 2.5 years

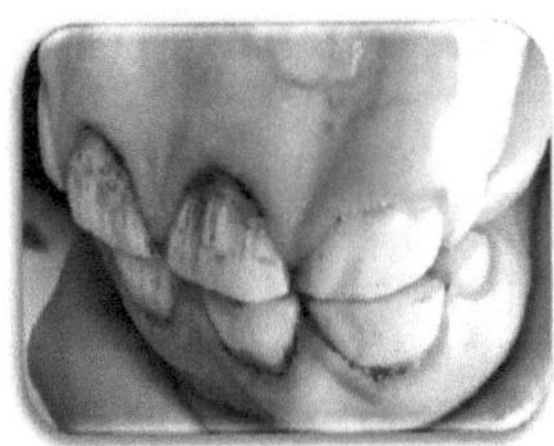

	Presence of: -First temporary incisor: present reaching shaving at the point of moulting. -Second temporary incisor: present and reaching shaving. -Third incisor: present and reaching shaving. At this stage of two and a half years the moulting of the first incisors occurs and we can observe the gum inflamed.

Stage 7 (36 months): 3 years

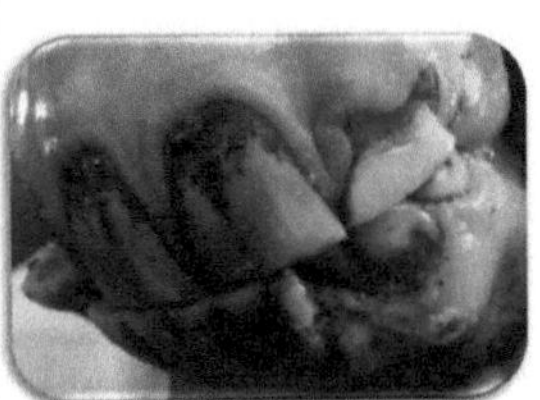

	Presence of: -First incisor: first permanent incisors present, reaching shaving.-Second incisor: Temporary teeth present. -Third incisor: temporary teeth present At this stage we can observe only the first permanent incisors present and reaching shaving, the second and third incisors are still temporary.We can differentiate the temporary pieces by shape and colour.

Eighth stage (42 months): 3.5 years	
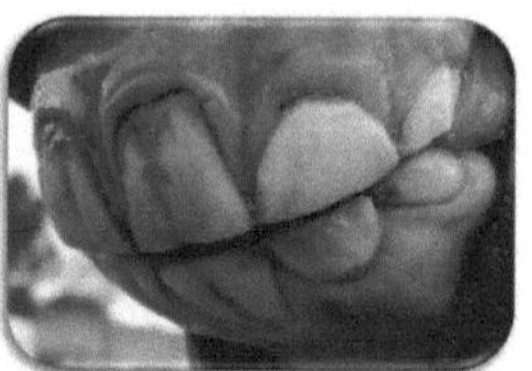	Presence of: -First incisor: first permanent incisors present, reaching shaving.-Second incisors: may be present newly erupted permanent or absent (in moult). -Third incisor: temporary teeth present.At this stage only the first permanent incisors are present and reaching shaving, the second incisors are in moult and the third incisors are still temporary. We can differentiate the temporary pieces by shape and colour.
Stage 9 (48 months): 4 years	
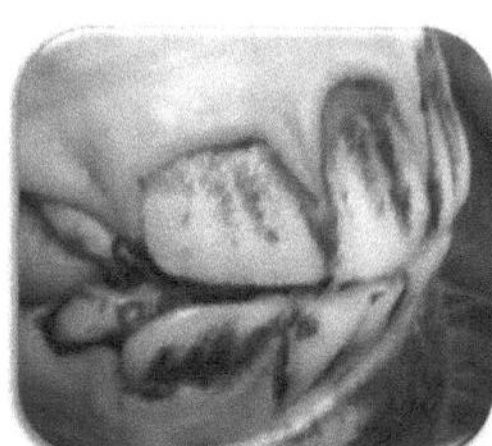	Presence of: -First incisor: first permanent incisors present, reaching shaving. -Second incisor: second permanent incisors present, reaching shaving. Third incisor: Temporary teeth present. At this stage of 4 years we can observe the first and second permanent incisors present and reaching shaving, while the third incisors are still temporary. We can differentiate the primary teeth by their shape and colour.
Stage ten (54 months): 4.5 years	
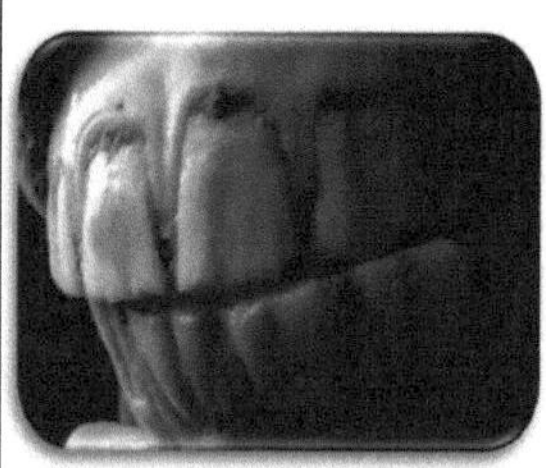	Presence of:-First incisor: first permanent incisors present, reaching shaving.-Second incisor: second permanent incisors present, reaching shaving.Third incisor: are in moultAt this stage of 4 and a half years we can observe the first and second permanent incisors present and reaching shaving, while the third incisors are in moult and about to fall out. We can observe the inflammation of the gums of the third incisors and the excessive wear of these indicating that they are about to fall out to be replaced by the permanent ones.
Stage 11 (60 months): 5 years	

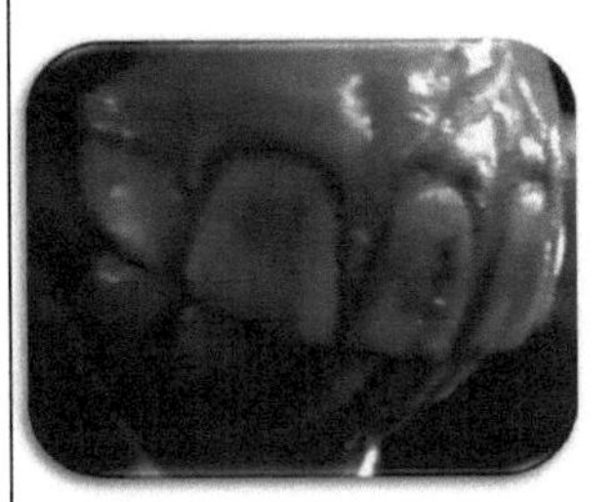

Presence of:
-First incisor: first permanent incisors present, reaching shaving.
-Second incisor: second permanent incisors present, reaching shaving.
-Third incisor: third permanent incisors present, reaching shaving.
At this stage of 5 years we can observe the first, second and third permanent incisors present and reaching shaving.
The mouth is said to be made up because it has all its permanent and shaved teeth.

CHAPTER VI

TABULATOR

Table 8. Age tabulator.

Temporary teeth				Permanent teeth		Incisors		
Months	Years	Eruption	Shaving	Muda	Shaving	First	Seconds	Third parties
	0 days	1T				1T		
2	2 months	1T					1T	
6	6 months	1T						1T
12	1 year		2T			2T		
18	1 year and a half		2T			2T	2T	
24	2 years		2T			2T	2T	2T
30	2 and a half years			3		3	2T	2T
36	3 years				4P	4P	2T	2T
42	3 and a half years			3	4P	4P	3	2T
48	4 years				3	3	3	2T
54	4 and a half years			3	4P	4P	4P	3
60	5 years				4P	4P	4P	4P

Eruption of primary teeth: 1T Shaving of primary teeth: 2T Molting: 3

Shaving permanent teeth: 4P

BIBLIOGRAPHY

Aguera Carmona, E., and Sandoval Juárez, J. 1999. Applied anatomy of the horse. Harcourt Brace.

Bennett, D. G. 2001. Bits and bitting: form and function. In Proceedings of the American Association of Equine Practitioners. Vol. 47, pp. 130-141.

Caldeira , R., Fausto Da Silva , M., Grave , J., Rosa, I., and Mendonca, H. 2002. Apontamentos de Exognosia. Lisbon: Faculdade de Medicina Veterinária, Universidade Técnica de Lisboa.

Dixon, P. M. 2002. The gross, histological, and ultrastructural anatomy of equine teeth and their relationship to disease. In Proceedings of the 49th Annual Convention of the American Association of Equine Practitioners. Vol. 48, pp. 421-437.

Dyce, K., Sack, W., and Wensing, C. 1991. Veterinary Anatomy. Argentina: Panamericana. Easley, J. 1996. Equine dental development and anatomy. In American Association of Equine Practitioners.

Esponda, V. 1981. Dental Anatomy. Sixth ed. Mexico: Print. Colección Textos Universitarios.

Foster, D. 1996. Nomenclature for equine dental anatomy based on the modified triadan system. 42nd Am. Assoc. Equine Practitioners Annual Convention, 18-319.

Frandson, R. D. 1988. Anatomy and physiology of domestic animals. mexico: Interamericana.

Frape, D. 1992. Nutrition and Feeding of the Horse. Spain: Acribia.

Frausto Da Silva, M., Gomes, T., Dias, A., Aquino, J., Mendes, L., Cavaco, J. 2003. Estimativa da idade dos equinos através do exame dentário. Rev. Port. Cienc. Vet., 103-110.

Getty, R. 1966. Atlas of applied veterinary anatomy (No. C SF 761. G4718 1966). Unión Tipográfica Editorial Hispanoamericana.

Gieche, J. M. 2007. How to assess equine oral health. How to assess equine oral health, 498-503.

Jones, S. 2005. Oral diseases. In: Reed, S.; Bayly, W.; Sellon, D. eds. Equine Internal Medicine. Vol. 2. 2nd ed. Argentina: Intermedica.

Kilic, S., Dixon, P. M., and Kempson, S. A. 1997. A light microscopic and ultrastructural examination of calcified dental tissues of horses: 3. Equine veterinary journal, 29(3), 206-212.

Kirkland, K. D., Baker, G. J., Eurell, J. A., and Losonsky, J. M. 1996. Effects of aging on the endodontic system, reserve crown, and roots of equine mandibular cheek teeth. American journal of veterinary research, 57(1), 31-38.

König, H. E., and Liebich, H. G. (2005). Anatomy of domestic animals: organs, circulatory system and nervous system. Ed. Médica Panamericana.

Lowder, M. Q., and Mueller, P. E. 1998. Dental embryology, anatomy, development, and aging. Veterinary clinics of North America: equine practice, 14(2), 227-245.

Marvin, G. 1992. Equine Dentistry. Argentina: Intermedica.

Mitchell, S. R., Kempson, S. A., and Dixon, P. M. 2003. Structure of peripheral cementum of normal equine cheek teeth. Journal of veterinary dentistry, 20(4), 199-208.

Morales, F. 1997. El Caballo. Marmor (Colombia), 356-358.

Pence, P. 2002. Equine Dentistry a practical guide. Philadelphia: Lippincott Williams & Wilkins.

Pimentel, L. 2007. Intraoral extraction techniques in standing horse. Pesq. Vet. Bras. 27, 57-58.

Richardson, J. 1997. Ageing horses-an illustrated guide. In Practice, 19(9), 486-489.

Richardson, J. D., Cripps, P. J., and Lane, J. G. 1995. An evaluation of the accuracy of ageing horses by their dentition: changes of dental morphology with age. Veterinary record, 137, 117-117.

Richardson, J. D., Lane, J. G., and Waldron, K. R. 1994. Is dentition an accurate indication of the age of a horse? The Veterinary Record, 135(2), 31-34.

Rucker, B. 2003. Diseases of the oral cavity and soft palate. Manual of Equine Gastroenterology. Ed. Intermedica (Argentina), 81-83.

Sandoval, J. 1976. Anatomy of the Horse. Head and Sense Organs. Volume III. Spain: Acribia.

Scoggins, R. D. 2001. Bits, bitting, and dentistry. Proceeding American Association of Equine Practitioners, 47, 138-141.

Scrutchfield, W. L., Schumacher, J., and Martin, M. T. 1996. Correction of abnormalities of the cheek teeth. American Association of Equine Practitioners (USA).

Scrutchfield, W. 2006. Wolf Teeth: How to Safely and Effectively Extract and Is It

Necessary. Am. Assoc. of Equine Practitioners.

Sisson, S., and Grossman, J. D. 2003. ANATOMY OF DOMESTIC ANIMALS .
Barcelona: MASSON .

Toit, N. 2006. Gross Equine Dentition and Their Supporting Structures. Am. Assoc. of
Equine Practitioners.

Townsend, N. B., Dixon, P. M., and Barakzai, S. Z. 2008. Evaluation of the long-term
oral consequences of equine exodontia in 50 horses. The Veterinary Journal, 178(3),
419-424.

Tremaine, H. 1997. Dental care in horses. In Practice, 19(4), 186-199.

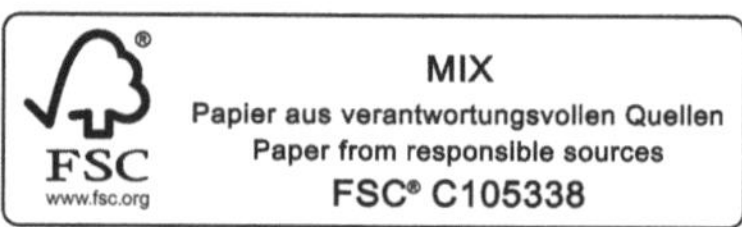

Printed by Books on Demand GmbH, Norderstedt / Germany